Copyright © 2017 by Melanie White

All rights reserved.

Published by Melanie White, www.downsizeme.net.au

Cover design and photography by Jennifer Akerstrom

Disclaimer:

This recipe book is designed to accompany the Downsize Me Program. For more information on this program, visit www.downsizeme.net.au.

The recipes and information in this book are provided for interest and educational purposes only.

Individual nutritional needs vary considerably. This book is not intended to provide prescriptive medical or dietary advice.

About this recipe book

My name is Melanie White.

I help determined women like you to create a healthier relationship with food and your body.

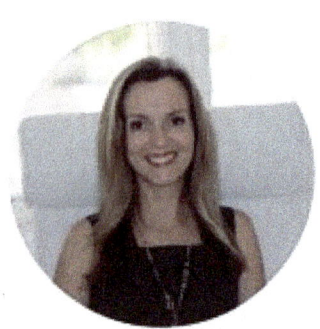

This Healthy Plant-Based Ice Cream recipe book is exactly what you need to make healthier choices.

Maybe you want to lose weight.

Maybe you have health conditions you're managing and can't eat certain things.

Maybe you're a vegan.

Or maybe, you just want to make healthier meals more often.

In any case, this recipe book is for you if your goal is to:

- ✓ Avoid added cane sugar
- ✓ Avoid thickeners, emulsifiers and preservatives
- ✓ Eat whole foods instead of processed, empty calories
- ✓ Improve your digestion and immunity
- ✓ Lose weight more easily
- ✓ Avoid animal products
- ✓ Create healthier, more nutrient-rich meals
- ✓ Feel good after eating ice cream
- ✓ Take control of your health.

When you have healthy options for those delicious treats you love, you'll experience total food freedom, without guilt, and you'll NEVER feel like you're missing out.

I hope you love this recipe book!

Best wishes

Melanie

Co-Founder, Downsize Me

www.downsizeme.net.au

About plant-based ice cream

Traditional ice cream is simply frozen custard. It's rich, creamy texture comes from fat (milk, cream, eggs) and sugar (cane sugar, fruit).

To get the same experience with whole plant foods, it's important that your plant-based ice cream contains natural fats, sugars and 'mouth feel' properties that are like traditional ice cream.

Some recipes in this book are high in fat. Some are high in carbohydrates and sugars. They may be like regular ice cream in terms of fat, sugar and calories.

The texture and consistency of these ice creams may vary and may be different from traditional ice creams. Some are more like sorbet, or ice confection….but they are quality tested, and similar enough that you will enjoy these delicious, healthy frozen desserts.

Hints and Tips for Ice Cream Success

Here's how to get the best results with plant-based ice cream.

- ✓ Coconut cream is creamier than coconut milk
- ✓ Our tasters voted the coconut and cashew-based ice creams to be most like traditional ice cream
- ✓ The coconut recipes use a 400mL can of coconut cream:
    - Of which about 300mL of coconut cream, and
    - Of which about 100mL of coconut milk
    - the nutritional breakdowns for each recipe are based on those portions
- ✓ You can pour ice cream mixes into icy-pole moulds
- ✓ Maple syrup can be substituted with honey, stevia, agave or rice malt syrup if desired…or omitted entirely. Taste the unfrozen mixture before adding.
- ✓ Experiment with other toppings and flavours!
- ✓ Where recipes call for dates, fresh dates are preferable to dried dates - the mix will be smoother.
- ✓ Dates can be replaced with a sweetener as listed above.

- ✓ These ice creams are best served immediately but can be kept in a sealed container or icy-pole mould in the freezer for 7 - 14 days.
- ✓ Plant-based ice creams are very firm when frozen - most need 5 – 10 minutes thawing time before serving.
- ✓ All these recipes are CHURN-FREE, BUT, you can use your ice cream maker for all of them. Simply:
    - follow the recipe, but
    - don't freeze any ingredients, and
    - then follow your ice cream maker's instructions.
- ✓ If using a Thermomix/high-speed blender, you can use pre-frozen ingredients.
- ✓ If using a food processor or normal blender, blend raw ingredients, then freeze.

Table of Contents

Avocado base 1
Matcha Green Tea 2
Mint Choc Chip 3
Pistachio 4
Rich Chocolate 5
Cashew base 6
Chai Cashew 7
Toasted Hazelnut and Coconut 8
Vanilla 9
Coconut base 10
Chocolate 11
Cinnamon Scroll 12
Coffee 13
Ginger and Cinnamon 14
Lemon 15
Rum and Raisin Vanilla Bean 16
Salted Caramel 17
Vanilla Bean 18
Fruit base 19
Banana 20
Berry Ice Cream 21
Choc banana ice cream 22
Chocolate Coconut 23
Mango 24
Orange 25
Peanut butter thunk 26
Strawberry Basil Ice cream 27
Tropical Sorbet 28
Toppings and Flavours 29
Berry Coulis 30
Caramel Sauce 31
Caramel Sauce (Creamy) 32
Chocolate Sauce 33
Peanut Butter Sauce 34
Strawberry Basil Sauce 35

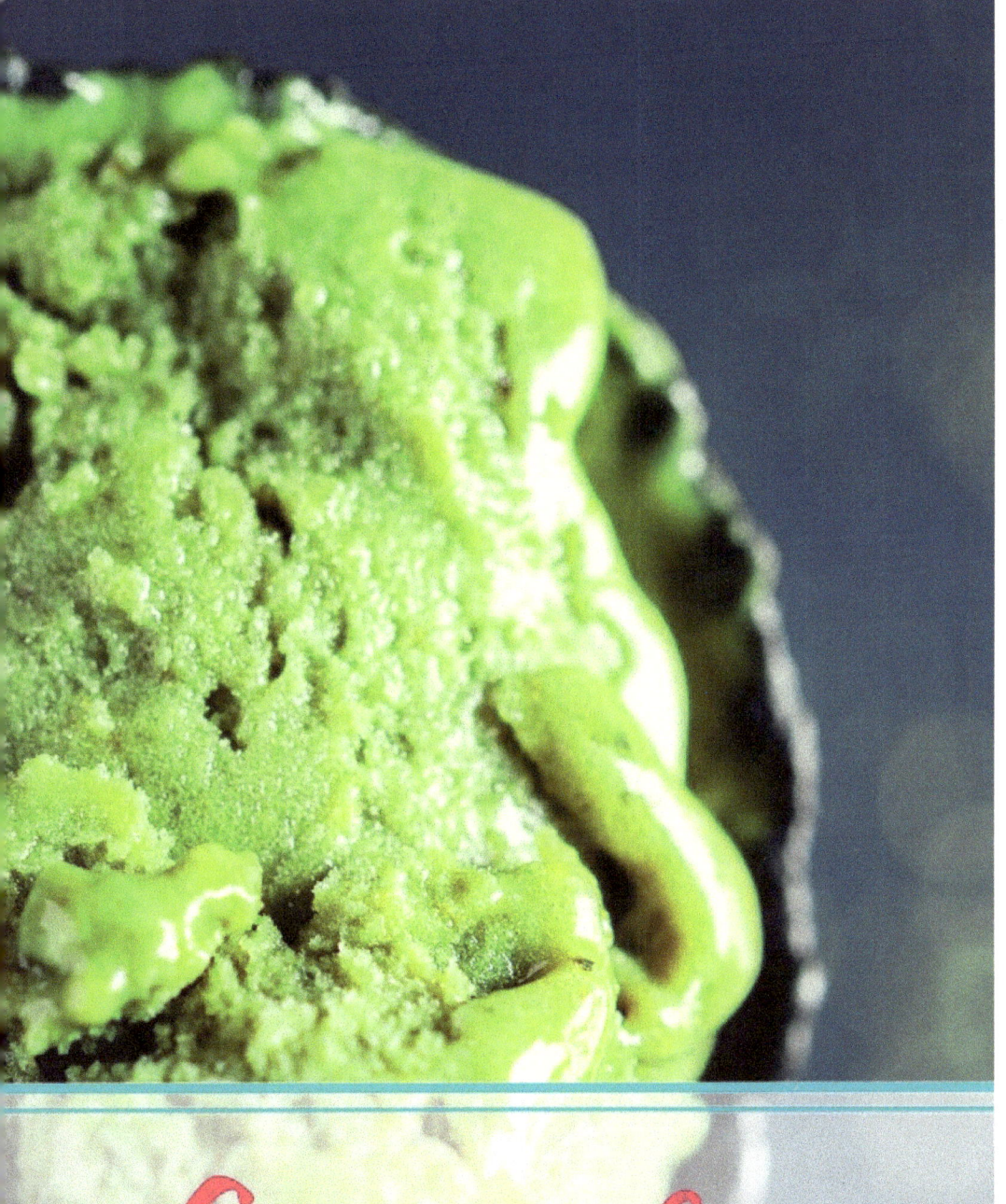

Matcha Green Tea

2 small avocadoes

1 cup coconut cream

2 tbsp honey

1 cup spinach leaves, stems removed

3 tsp matcha green tea powder

1 pinch salt

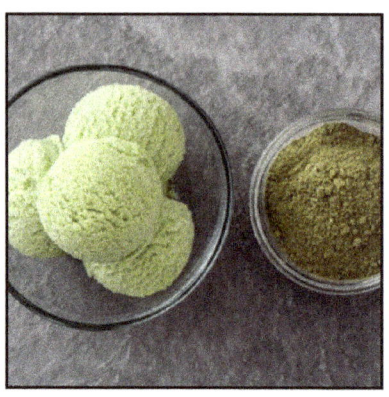

Procedure

1. Blend all ingredients in a Thermomix or high-speed blender until smooth.
2. Transfer to a silicone loaf pan or a baking paper-lined loaf tin.
3. Freeze for at least 3 hours and allow to thaw for a few minutes if required before serving.

Servings: 8

Preparation Time: 10 minutes

Inactive Time: 3 hours

Total Time: 3 hours and 10 minutes

Nutrition Facts

Nutrition (per serving): 198 calories, 17.8g total fat, 0mg cholesterol, 10.4mg sodium, 365.1mg potassium, 10.7g carbohydrates, 4.4g fibre, 4.7g sugar, 2.5g protein.

Mint Choc Chip

2 whole avocadoes
1 large banana
1/2 cup coconut cream
1 pinch salt
8 drops peppermint oil
2 tbsp mint leaves
1 tbsp maple syrup (pure)
1 tbsp cacao nibs

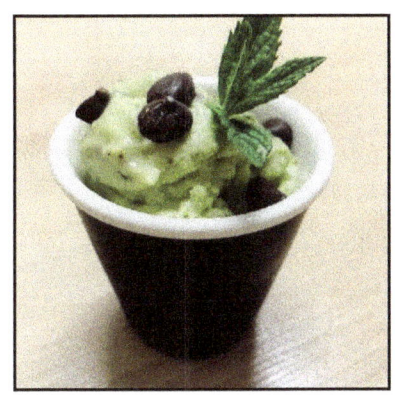

Procedure

1. Peel and slice the banana, freeze overnight in an airtight container.
2. Blend frozen banana with all other ingredients except the cacao nibs in a Thermomix or high-powered blender until smooth.
3. Add the cacao nibs at the end and stir through (or 10s on Reverse Sp 3 in Thermomix).
4. Transfer to a silicon loaf pan or baking paper-lined loaf tin.
5. Freeze for at least 2 hours and allow to thaw for a few minutes if required, before serving.

Servings: 4

Preparation Time: 10 minutes

Inactive Time: 3 hours

Total Time: 3 hours and 10 minutes

Nutrition Facts

Nutrition (per serving): 323 calories, 26.8g total fat, 0mg cholesterol, 82.1mg sodium, 748.1mg potassium, 23.4g carbohydrates, 9.5g fibre, 8.2g sugar, 4g protein.

Healthy Plant Based Ice Cream Avocado base

Pistachio

1 whole avocado
1/2 cup rice milk
1/2 large banana
2 tbsp maple syrup
1/2 cup spinach leaves
1/2 tsp almond extract
1 tsp lime juice
1/4 cup pistachio raw nuts, roughly chopped

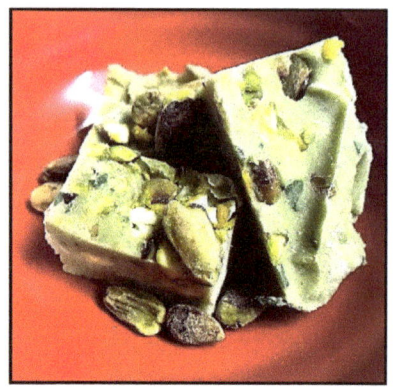

Procedure

1. Blend all ingredients except pistachios on high-powered in a Thermomix or food processor until smooth and lump-free.
2. Stir through crumbled pistachios, reserving 1 tbsp to sprinkle over the top.
3. Transfer to a silicone loaf pan or baking paper-lined loaf pan and top with reserved pistachios.
4. Freeze for at least 3 hours and allow to thaw for a few minutes if required before serving.

Servings: 6

Preparation Time: 10 minutes

Inactive Time: 3 hours

Total Time: 3 hours and 10 minutes

Nutrition Facts

Nutrition (per serving): 123 calories, 7.5g total fat, 0mg cholesterol, 20.9mg sodium, 284.7mg potassium, 13.7g carbohydrates, 3.1g fibre, 7.1g sugar, 2g protein.

Rich Chocolate

1 whole avocado
1/2 large banana
1/2 cup coconut cream
2 tbsp maple syrup
1 tsp vanilla extract
2 tbsp cacao powder

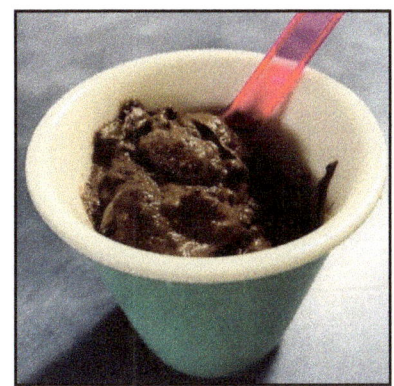

Procedure

1. Blend all ingredients in a Thermomix or high-powered blender until smooth.
2. Transfer to a silicon loaf pan or a baking paper-lined loaf tin and freeze for at least 3 hours.
3. Allow to thaw for a few minutes before serving.

Servings: 6

Preparation Time: 10 minutes

Inactive Time: 3 hours

Total Time: 3 hours and 10 minutes

Nutrition Facts

Nutrition (per serving): 153 calories, 12.1g total fat, 0mg cholesterol, 4.5mg sodium, 283mg potassium, 11.6g carbohydrates, 3.6g fibre, 6.2g sugar, 2.1g protein.

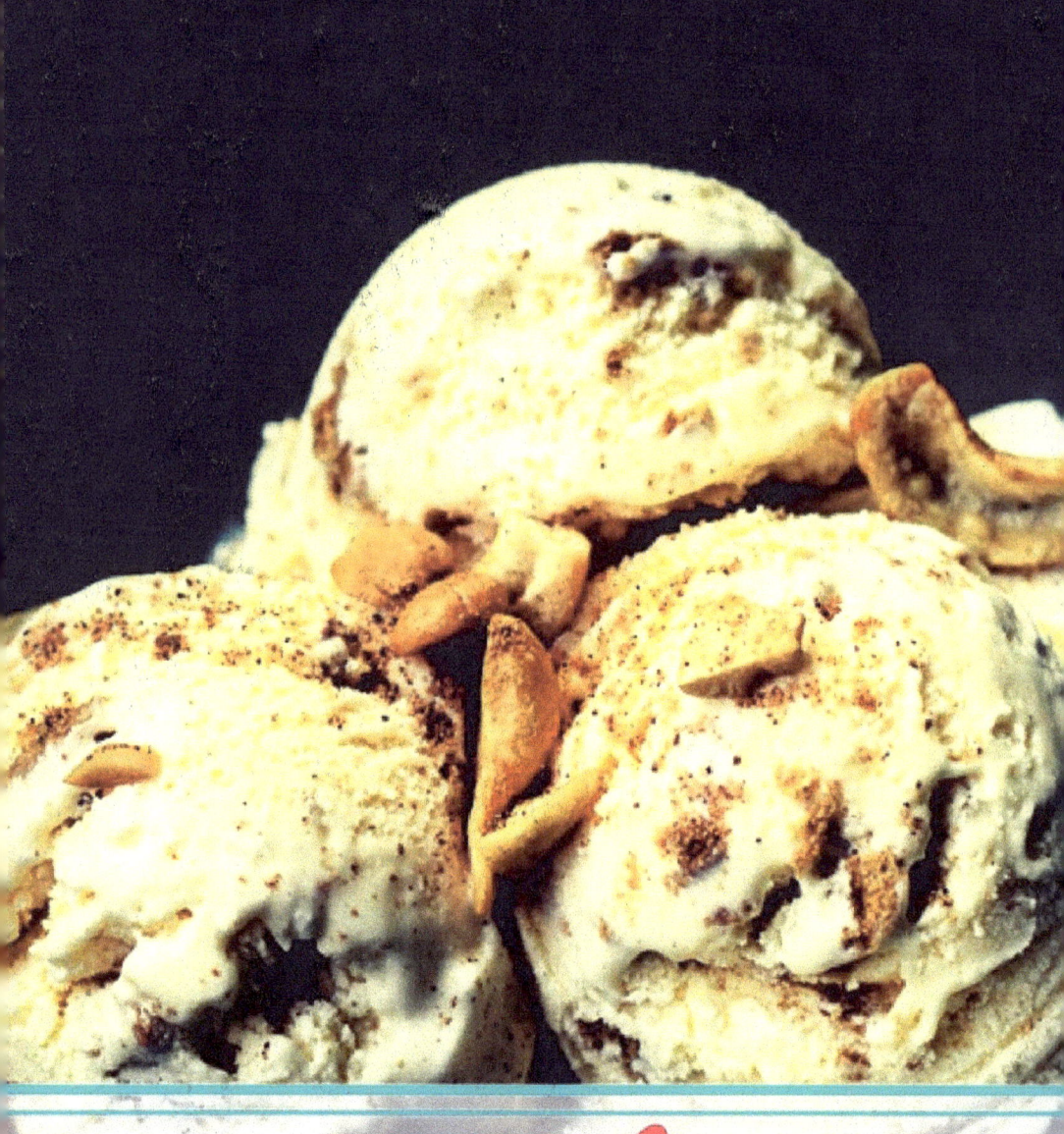

Chai Cashew

1 cup cashews
1 tbsp coconut oil
3 tbsp honey
1/2 cup rice milk
2 Bengal spice or chai tea bags in 1/2 cup boiling water
1 tsp vanilla extract
1 tsp mixed spice

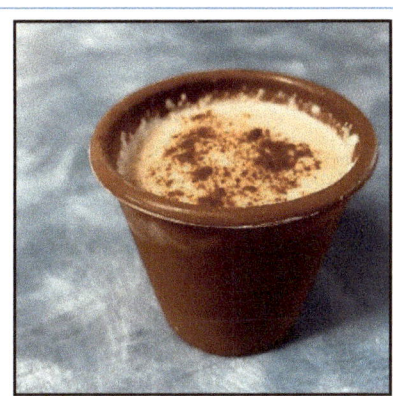

Procedure

1. Cover cashews with water and soak overnight (> 24 hours), then drain and rinse well.
2. Steep tea bags in boiling water for 5 - 10 minutes; remove teabags.
3. Blend cashews well, until very smooth, in a Thermomix or high-speed blender.
4. Add Bengal spice or chai tea and remaining ingredients and blend until smooth.
5. Transfer to a silicon loaf pan or baking paper-lined loaf tin.
6. Freeze at least 6 hours or overnight, and thaw for a few minutes if required before serving.

Servings: 6

Preparation Time: 15 minutes

Inactive Time: 24 hours

Total Time: 24 hours and 15 minutes

Nutrition Facts

Nutrition (per serving): 204 calories, 13.5g total fat, 0mg cholesterol, 20mg sodium, 182mg potassium, 19g carbohydrates, <1g fibre, 11g sugar, 4.7g protein.

Toasted Hazelnut and Coconut

1 cup cashews
1 tbsp coconut oil
3 tbsp maple syrup
½ tsp ground cinnamon
4 dates, pitted (fresh are best)
1 cup rice milk
1 tsp vanilla extract
1/4 cup hazelnuts
2 tbsp coconut flakes

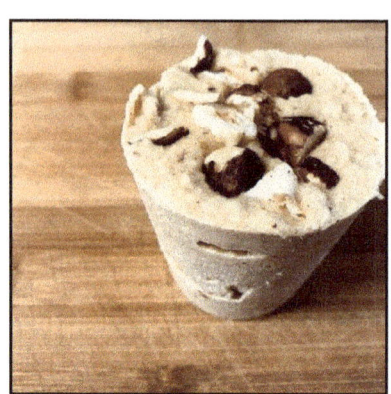

Procedure

1. Cover cashews with water and soak overnight (> 24 hours), then drain and rinse well.
2. Cover the dates with boiling water and soak for 5 - 10 minutes, drain well and remove skins.
3. Add coconut oil, maple syrup, soaked dates, milk, cinnamon and vanilla extract, then blend until smooth and creamy.
4. Transfer cashew mix to a silicon loaf pan or paper-lined tin.
5. Roughly chop hazelnuts and dry toast with coconut flakes in a non-stick pan on medium heat.
6. Sprinkle the ice cream with about 3/4 of the hazelnut and coconut flakes, stir through carefully, keep the rest aside.
7. Freeze for at least 6 hours or overnight, thaw for 10 minutes, then top with reserved hazelnuts and coconut flakes.

Servings: 8

Preparation Time: 20 minutes

Inactive Time: 24 hours

Total Time: 24 hours and 20 minutes

Nutrition Facts

Nutrition (per serving): 216 calories, 12.8g total fat, 0mg cholesterol, 27mg sodium, 252mg potassium, 24g carbohydrates, 2g fibre, 15.3g sugar, 4.4g protein.

Healthy Plant Based Ice Cream　　　　Cashew base

Vanilla

1 cup cashews
1 banana
1/2 cup coconut cream
3 tbsp maple syrup (optional)
1 tsp vanilla extract

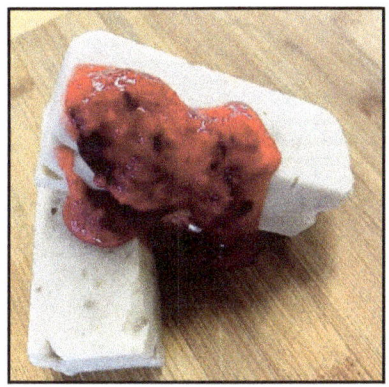

Procedure

1. Cover cashews with water and soak overnight (> 24 hours), then drain and rinse well.
2. Blend cashews well, until very smooth, in a Thermomix or high-speed blender.
3. Add remaining ingredients and blend until smooth.
4. Transfer to a silicon loaf pan or baking paper-lined loaf tin.
5. Freeze at least 6 hours or overnight, and thaw for a few minutes if required before serving.

Servings: 8

Preparation Time: 10 minutes

Inactive Time: 24 hours

Total Time: 24 hours and 10 minutes

Nutrition Facts

Nutrition (per serving): 187 calories, 13.5g total fat, 0mg cholesterol, 3.9mg sodium, 242mg potassium, 15.1g carbohydrates, 1.3g fibre, 8.1g sugar, 4.1g protein.

Recipe Tips

This is delicious with strawberry basil sauce (pictured).

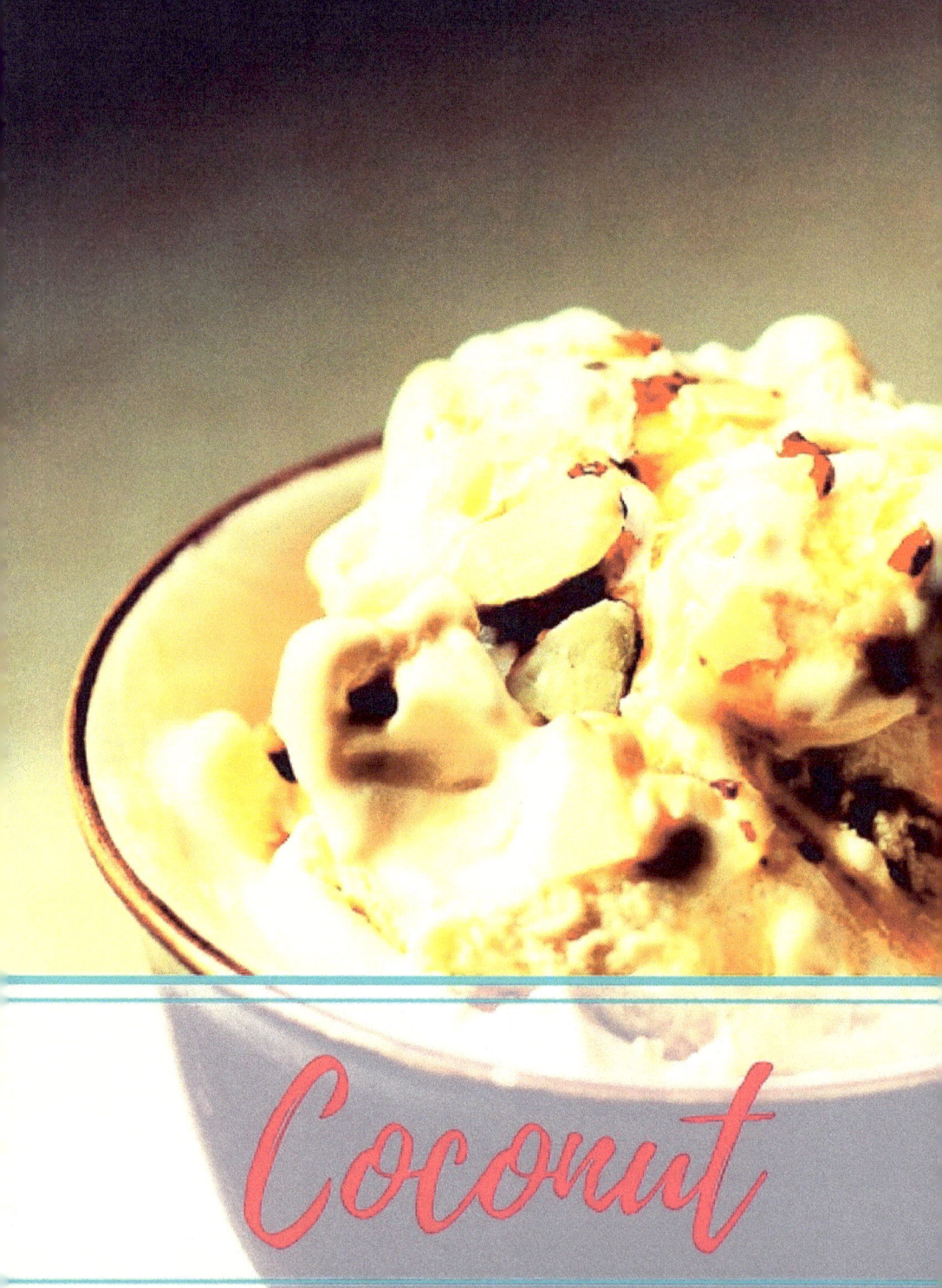

Chocolate

300 mL coconut cream
100 mL coconut milk
6 dates, pitted (fresh are best)
1/2 cup rice milk
2 tbsp cacao
1 tsp vanilla extract
1 pinch salt

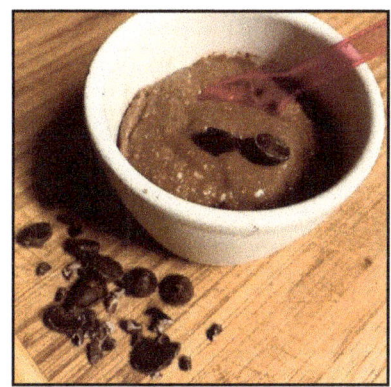

Procedure

1. Pour the coconut cream into a snaplock bag, ice cube tray or sealed container and freeze overnight.
2. Cover the dates with boiling water and soak for 5 - 10 minutes, drain well and remove skins.
3. Blend the coconut cream with dates and remaining ingredients until smooth.
4. Transfer to a silicon loaf pan or baking paper-lined loaf tin and freeze for at least 30 minutes.
5. Allow to thaw for a few minutes before serving if required, or store in a well-sealed container in the freezer.

Servings: 8

Preparation Time: 15 minutes

Inactive Time: 24 hours

Total Time: 24 hours and 15 minutes

Nutrition Facts

Nutrition (per serving): 213 calories, 16g total fat, 0mg cholesterol, 17.8mg sodium, 277.6mg potassium, 18.7g carbohydrates, 2.5g fibre, 12.5g sugar, 2.4g protein.

Recipe Tips

Stir through chocolate chips or cacao nibs if desired before freezing.

Cinnamon Scroll

300 mL coconut cream
100 mL coconut milk
1/2 cup almond butter
6 dates, pitted (fresh are best)
1 pinch salt
1 tsp vanilla extract
4 tbsp maple syrup
3 tsp cinnamon

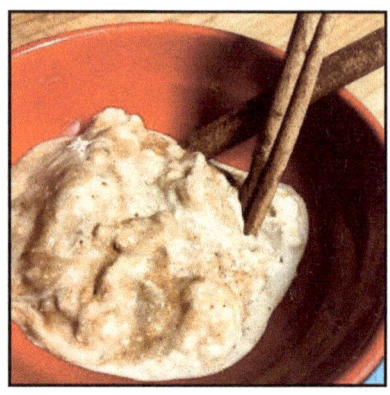

Procedure

1. Pour the coconut milk and cream into a snaplock bag, ice cube tray or sealed container and freeze overnight.
2. Transfer frozen coconut milk and cream to a Thermomix or high-speed blender and add almond butter, almond milk, salt and vanilla extract and 5 of the dates; blend until smooth.
3. Transfer to a silicon loaf pan or baking paper-lined loaf tin and place in the freezer to keep cold.
4. Blend the remaining date with maple syrup and cinnamon; add a little hot water if required to get a smooth consistency.
5. Swirl cinnamon sauce through the ice cream with a knife.
6. Return to freezer to harden if required, or serve immediately, or store in a well-sealed container in the freezer.

Servings: 10

Preparation Time: 10 minutes

Inactive Time: 24 hours

Total Time: 24 hours and 10 minutes

Nutrition Facts

Nutrition (per serving): 185 calories, 12.7g total fat, 0mg cholesterol, 37.7mg sodium, 244.5mg potassium, 19.5g carbohydrates, 2.1g fibre, 15.4g sugar, 1.6g protein.

Coffee

300 mL coconut cream
100 mL coconut milk
1 tsp vanilla extract
3 tbsp maple syrup
1/2 cup espresso coffee

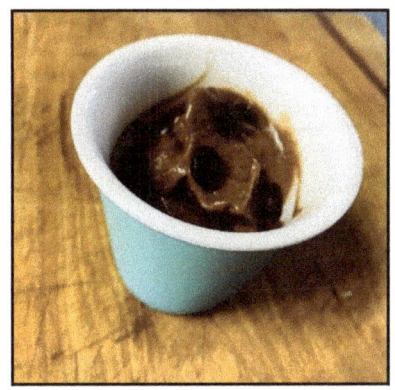

Procedure

1. Pour the coconut cream into a snaplock bag, ice cube tray or sealed container and freeze overnight.
2. Pour the espresso into an ice cube tray and freeze overnight.
3. Blend all ingredients in a Thermomix or high-speed blender until smooth.
4. Freeze briefly to harden if required, or serve immediately, or store in a well-sealed container in the freezer.

Servings: 8

Preparation Time: 15 minutes

Inactive Time: 24 hours

Total Time: 24 hours and 15 minutes

Nutrition Facts

Nutrition (per serving): 173 calories, 15.7g total fat, 0mg cholesterol, 7.9mg sodium, 200.6mg potassium, 8.8g carbohydrates, <1g fibre, 5.2g sugar, 1.6g protein.

Recipe Tips

Stir through chocolate chips if desired before freezing, or sprinkle with chocolate-coated coffee beans.
Fresh dates are preferable if available.

Ginger and Cinnamon

300 mL coconut cream

100 mL coconut milk

1 pinch salt

3 tbsp maple syrup or honey (if desired)

1 tsp vanilla extract

1 tsp ginger-root; fresh; minced

2 tsp cinnamon

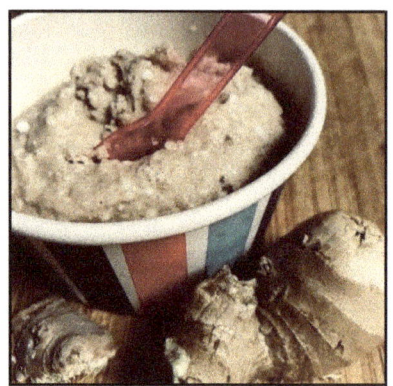

Procedure

1. Pour the coconut cream into a snaplock bag, ice cube tray or sealed container and freeze overnight.
2. Transfer frozen coconut cream to a Thermomix or high-speed blender and add remaining ingredients; blend until smooth.
3. Serve immediately, or store in a well-sealed container in the freezer.

Servings: 10

Preparation Time: 10 minutes

Inactive Time: 24 hours

Total Time: 24 hours and 10 minutes

Nutrition Facts

Nutrition (per serving): 137 calories, 12.5g total fat, 0mg cholesterol, 32.8mg sodium, 137mg potassium, 7g carbohydrates, <1g fibre, 4g sugar, 1.3g protein.

Lemon

300 mL coconut cream
100 mL coconut milk
1 pinch salt
2 tbsp lemon juice
1 tbsp lemon zest
4 drops lemon oil or other citrus oil (optional)
1 tbsp honey, or to taste

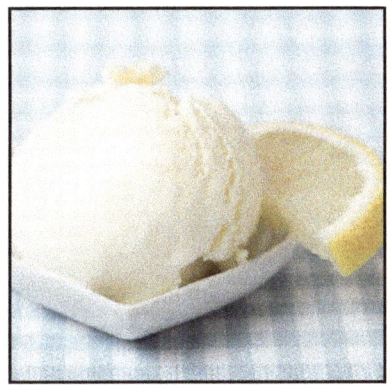

Procedure

1. Pour the coconut cream into a snaplock bag, ice cube tray or sealed container and freeze overnight.
2. Pour the lemon juice into an ice cube tray and freeze overnight.
3. Transfer frozen coconut cream and lemon juice to a Thermomix or high-speed blender and add remaining ingredients; blend until smooth.
4. Serve immediately, or store in a well-sealed container in the freezer.

Servings: 6

Preparation Time: 10 minutes

Inactive Time: 24 hours

Total Time: 24 hours and 10 minutes

Nutrition Facts

Nutrition (per serving): 211 calories, 20.9g total fat, 0mg cholesterol, 52.7mg sodium, 210.4mg potassium, 7.7g carbohydrates, 1.2g fibre, 3g sugar, 2.1g protein.

Rum and Raisin Vanilla Bean

300 mL coconut cream
100 mL coconut milk
2 tbsp dark or spiced rum
2 tbsp raisins
6 dates, pitted (fresh are best)
1/2 cup rice milk
1 tsp vanilla extract
1 whole vanilla bean, scraped
1 pinch salt

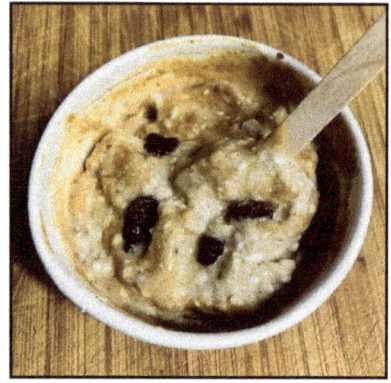

Procedure

1. Pour the coconut cream into a snaplock bag, ice cube tray or sealed container and freeze overnight.
2. Place the raisins into a small jar or cup and pour over rum; cover and soak overnight.
3. Cover the dates with boiling water and soak for 5 - 10 minutes, drain well and remove skins.
4. Blend the frozen coconut cream with dates, milk, vanilla, vanilla bean seeds from the pod and salt until smooth.
5. Strain the rum out of the raisins and set raisins aside.
6. Pour rum into the ice cream mix and pulse to combine.
7. Transfer the ice cream to a silicon loaf pan or paper-lined tin.
8. Stir the raisins through the ice cream mix with a knife, then transfer to the freezer until desired hardness is achieved.

Servings: 8

Preparation Time: 20 minutes

Inactive Time: 24 hours

Total Time: 24 hours and 20 minutes

Nutrition Facts

Nutrition (per serving): 224 calories, 15.8g total fat, 0mg cholesterol, 17.7mg sodium, 294.6mg potassium, 20.2g carbohydrates, 2.1g fibre, 13.8g sugar, 2.1g protein.

Salted Caramel

300 mL coconut cream
100 mL coconut milk
1 banana
1 tsp tahini
1 pinch salt
6 dates, pitted (fresh are best)

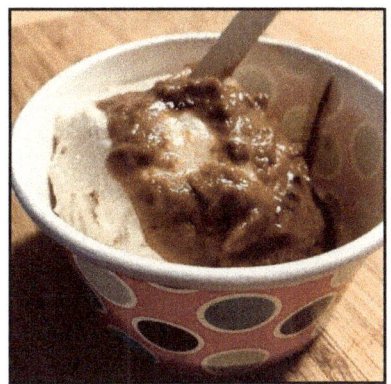

Procedure

1. Freeze the peeled, sliced banana and the coconut cream in two separate containers overnight.
2. Soak dates in boiling water for 5 - 10 minutes; remove skins.
3. Blend the frozen coconut cream and banana until smooth.
4. Transfer to a silicon loaf pan or baking paper-lined loaf tin and put into the freezer to keep cold.
5. Blend drained dates, salt and tahini until smooth & creamy.
6. Transfer the date mix (caramel) to a small, shallow bowl.
7. Remove the ice cream from the freezer and swirl the caramel into the ice cream with a silicon spatula.
8. Serve immediately, or freeze for 15 mins if required, or store in a well-sealed container in the freezer.

Servings: 8

Preparation Time: 15 minutes

Inactive Time: 24 hours

Total Time: 24 hours and 15 minutes

Nutrition Facts

Nutrition (per serving): 223 calories, 16.6g total fat, 0mg cholesterol, 41.1mg sodium, 337.2mg potassium, 20.6g carbohydrates, 2.6g fibre, 13.8g sugar, 2.4g protein.

Vanilla Bean

300 mL coconut cream
100 mL coconut milk
1 pinch salt
1 tbsp maple syrup or honey (if desired)
1 tsp vanilla extract
1 vanilla bean, split and scraped

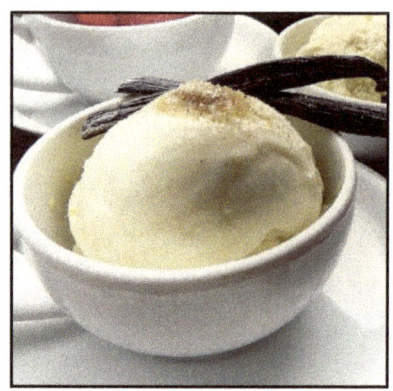

Procedure

1. Pour the coconut cream into a snaplock bag, ice cube tray or sealed container and freeze overnight.
2. Transfer frozen coconut cream to a Thermomix or high-speed blender and add remaining ingredients including scraped vanilla bean seeds; blend until smooth.
3. Serve immediately, or store in a well-sealed container in the freezer.

Servings: 6

Preparation Time: 5 minutes

Inactive Time: 24 hours

Total Time: 24 hours and 5 minutes

Nutrition Facts

Nutrition (per serving): 210 calories, 20.9g total fat, 0mg cholesterol, 52.9mg sodium, 209.8mg potassium, 6.6g carbohydrates, 1.1g fibre, 2.4g sugar, 2.1g protein.

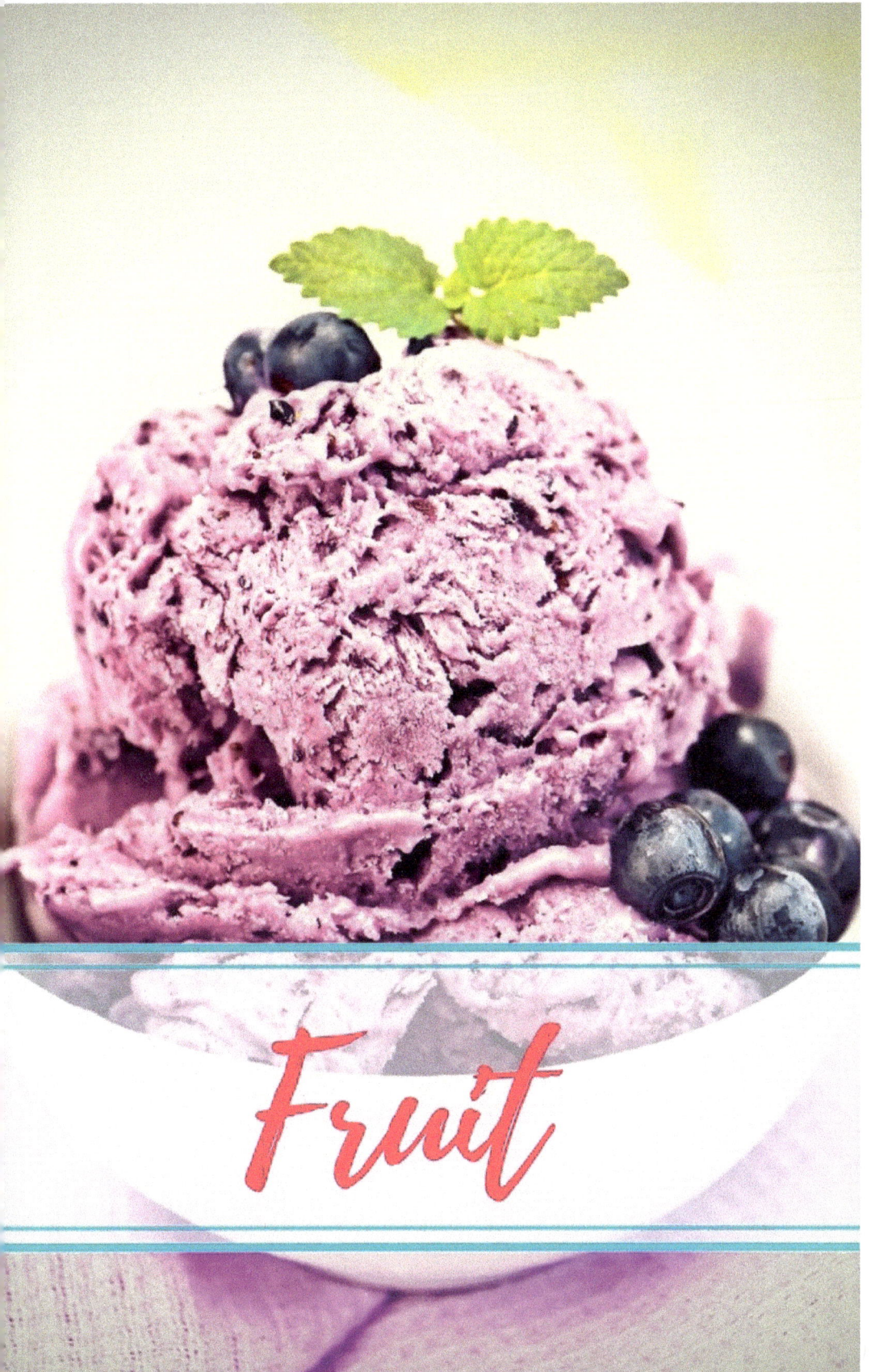

Banana

1 large banana

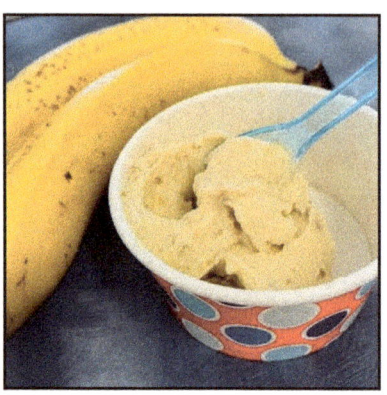

Procedure

1. Peel and chop the banana; freeze overnight in a sealed container.
2. Place frozen fruit in a Thermomix or high-powered blender and blend until smooth and creamy.
3. Serve immediately or store in a well-sealed container in the freezer.

Servings: 2

Preparation Time: 5 minutes

Inactive Time: 24 hours

Total Time: 24 hours and 5 minutes

Nutrition Facts

Nutrition (per serving): 61 calories, <1g total fat, 0mg cholesterol, <1mg sodium, 243.4mg potassium, 15.5g carbohydrates, 1.8g fibre, 8.3g sugar, <1g protein.

Recipe Tips

Unused portion can be frozen in a sealed container for up to 14 days. Allow 5 - 10 minutes to soften at room temperature before serving.

Berry Ice Cream

1 large banana

1 cup mixed berries (fresh or frozen)

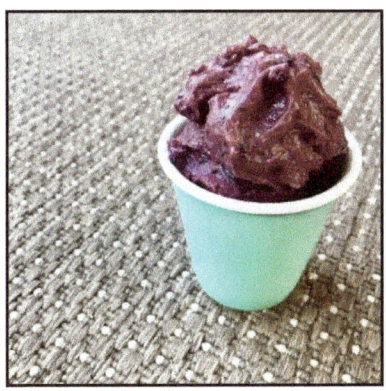

Procedure

1. Peel and chop the banana; freeze overnight in a sealed container.
2. If using fresh berries, place them in a sealed container and freeze overnight.
3. Place frozen fruit in a Thermomix or high-powered blender and blend until smooth and creamy.
4. Serve immediately or store in a well-sealed container in the freezer.

Servings: 2

Preparation Time: 5 minutes

Inactive Time: 24 hours

Total Time: 24 hours and 5 minutes

Nutrition Facts

Nutrition (per serving): 102 calories, <1g total fat, 0mg cholesterol, 1.4mg sodium, 299.3mg potassium, 26g carbohydrates, 3.5g fibre, 15.5g sugar, 1.3g protein.

Recipe Tips

Unused portion can be frozen in a sealed container for up to 14 days. Allow 5 - 10 minutes to soften at room temperature before serving.

Choc banana ice cream

2 large bananas
1 tsp vanilla extract
2 tbsp raw cacao powder

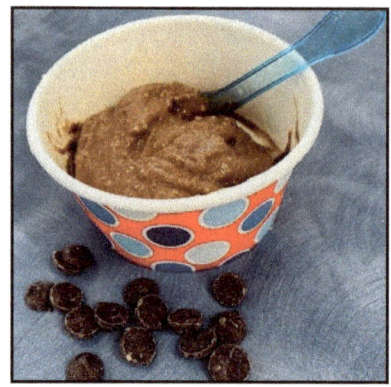

Procedure

1. Peel and chop the banana; freeze overnight in a sealed container.
2. Blend the banana, vanilla and cacao in a Thermomix or high-powered blender and blend until smooth and creamy.
3. Serve immediately or store in a well-sealed container in the freezer.

Servings: 4

Preparation Time: 5 minutes

Inactive Time: 24 hours

Total Time: 24 hours and 5 minutes

Nutrition Facts

Nutrition (per serving): 71 calories, <1g total fat, 0mg cholesterol, 1.4mg sodium, 245mg potassium, 16.2g carbohydrates, 2.7g fibre, 8.5g sugar, 1.6g protein.

Recipe Tips

Unused portion can be frozen in a sealed container for up to 14 days. Allow 5 - 10 minutes to soften at room temperature before serving.

Chocolate Coconut

2 large bananas
1.5 tbsp raw cacao powder
2 tbsp coconut cream
1 tsp vanilla extract
2 tbsp flaked coconut

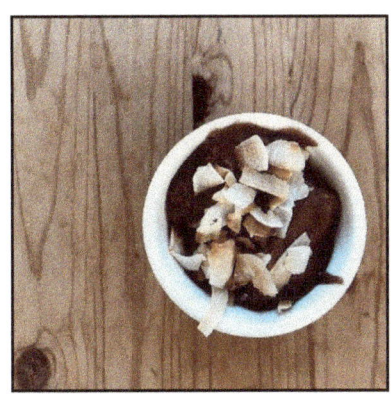

Procedure

1. Peel and chop the banana; freeze overnight in a container.
2. Pour the coconut cream into ice cube trays and freeze overnight.
3. Blend frozen banana, coconut cream, cacao and vanilla into a Thermomix or high-powered blender until creamy.
4. Add coconut flakes and stir through.
5. Serve immediately or store in a well-sealed container in the freezer.

Servings: 4

Preparation Time: 5 minutes

Inactive Time: 24 hours

Total Time: 24 hours and 5 minutes

Nutrition Facts

Nutrition (per serving): 104 calories, 3.7g total fat, 0mg cholesterol, 8.1mg sodium, 277.7mg potassium, 17.7g carbohydrates, 2.9g fibre, 9.3g sugar, 1.7g protein.

Recipe Tips

Unused portion can be frozen in a sealed container for up to 14 days. Allow 5 - 10 minutes to soften at room temperature before serving.

Mango

1 large mango

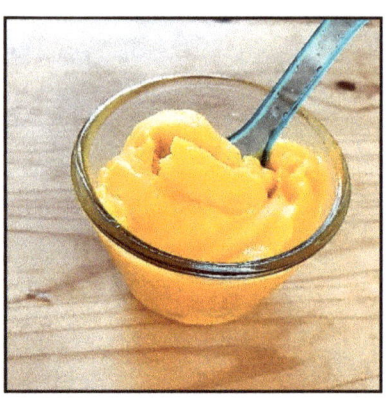

Procedure

1. Peel, de-seed and chop the mango; freeze overnight in a sealed container.
2. Place frozen fruit in a Thermomix or high-powered blender and blend until smooth and creamy.
3. Serve immediately or store in a well-sealed container in the freezer.

Servings: 2

Preparation Time: 5 minutes

Inactive Time: 24 hours

Total Time: 24 hours and 5 minutes

Nutrition Facts

Nutrition (per serving): 101 calories, <1g total fat, 0mg cholesterol, 1.7mg sodium, 282.2mg potassium, 25.2g carbohydrates, 2.7g fibre, 23g sugar, 1.4g protein.

Recipe Tips

Unused portion can be frozen in a sealed container for up to 14 days. Allow 5 - 10 minutes to soften at room temperature before serving.

Orange

2 large oranges

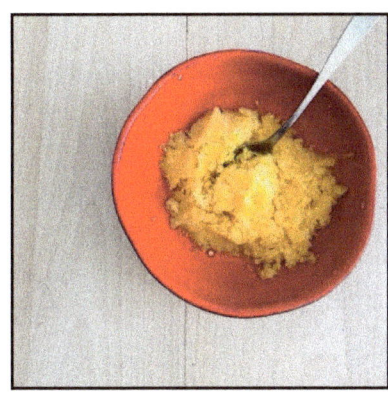

Procedure

1. Peel, de-seed and chop the orange; freeze overnight in a sealed container.
2. Place frozen fruit in a Thermomix or high-powered blender and blend until smooth and creamy.
3. Serve immediately or store in a well-sealed container in the freezer.

Servings: 2

Preparation Time: 5 minutes

Inactive Time: 24 hours

Total Time: 24 hours and 5 minutes

Nutrition Facts

Nutrition (per serving): 86 calories, <1g total fat, 0mg cholesterol, 0mg sodium, 333mg potassium, 21.6g carbohydrates, 4.4g fibre, 17.2g sugar, 1.7g protein.

Recipe Tips

Unused portion can be frozen in a sealed container for up to 14 days. Allow 5 - 10 minutes to soften at room temperature before serving.

Peanut butter thunk

1 large banana

2 tbsp peanut butter (sugar free)

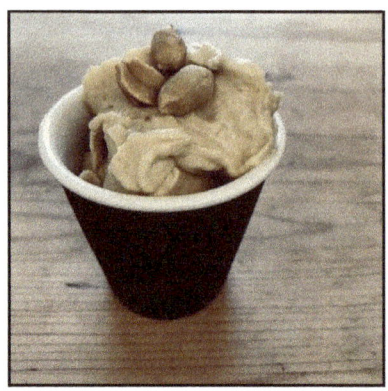

Procedure

1. Peel and chop the banana; freeze overnight in a sealed container.
2. Place frozen banana and peanut butter into a Thermomix or high-powered blender and blend until smooth and creamy.
3. Serve immediately or store in a well-sealed container in the freezer.

Servings: 4

Preparation Time: 5 minutes

Inactive Time: 24 hours

Total Time: 24 hours and 5 minutes

Nutrition Facts

Nutrition (per serving): 78 calories, 4.2g total fat, 0mg cholesterol, 37.3mg sodium, 174mg potassium, 9.3g carbohydrates, 1.4g fibre, 4.9g sugar, 2.4g protein.

Recipe Tips

Unused portion can be frozen in a sealed container for up to 14 days. Allow 5 - 10 minutes to soften at room temperature before serving.

Strawberry Basil Ice cream

1 large banana

1 punnet strawberries, washed and stemmed

1 sprig basil leaves

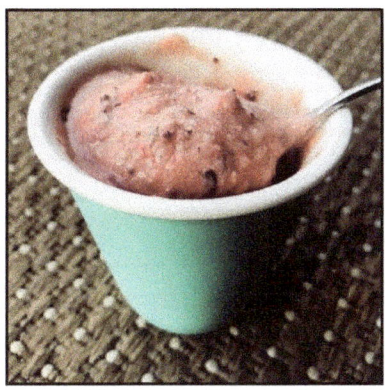

Procedure

1. Peel and chop the banana; freeze overnight with the washed and hulled strawberries, in a sealed container.
2. Place frozen fruit and basil leaves into a Thermomix or high-powered blender and blend until smooth and creamy.
3. Serve immediately or store in a well-sealed container in the freezer.

Servings: 2

Preparation Time: 5 minutes

Inactive Time: 24 hours

Total Time: 24 hours and 5 minutes

Nutrition Facts

Nutrition (per serving): 85 calories, <1g total fat, 0mg cholesterol, 1.5mg sodium, 363.4mg potassium, 21.4g carbohydrates, 3.3g fibre, 12g sugar, 1.3g protein.

Recipe Tips

Unused portion can be frozen in a sealed container for up to 14 days. Allow 5 - 10 minutes to soften at room temperature before serving.

Tropical Sorbet

1 large banana
1 1/2 mango, peeled, seeded and chopped

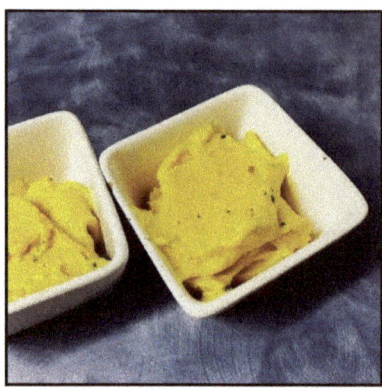

Procedure

1. Peel and chop the banana and mango; freeze overnight in a sealed container.
2. Place frozen fruit in a Thermomix or high-powered blender and blend until smooth and creamy.
3. Serve immediately or store in a well-sealed container in the freezer.

Servings: 4

Preparation Time: 5 minutes

Inactive Time: 24 hours

Total Time: 24 hours and 5 minutes

Nutrition Facts

Nutrition (per serving): 81 calories, <1g total fat, 0mg cholesterol, 1.2mg sodium, 262.8mg potassium, 20.4g carbohydrates, 2.2g fibre, 15.6g sugar, 1.1g protein.

Recipe Tips

Unused portion can be frozen in a sealed container for up to 14 days. Allow 5 - 10 minutes to soften at room temperature before serving.

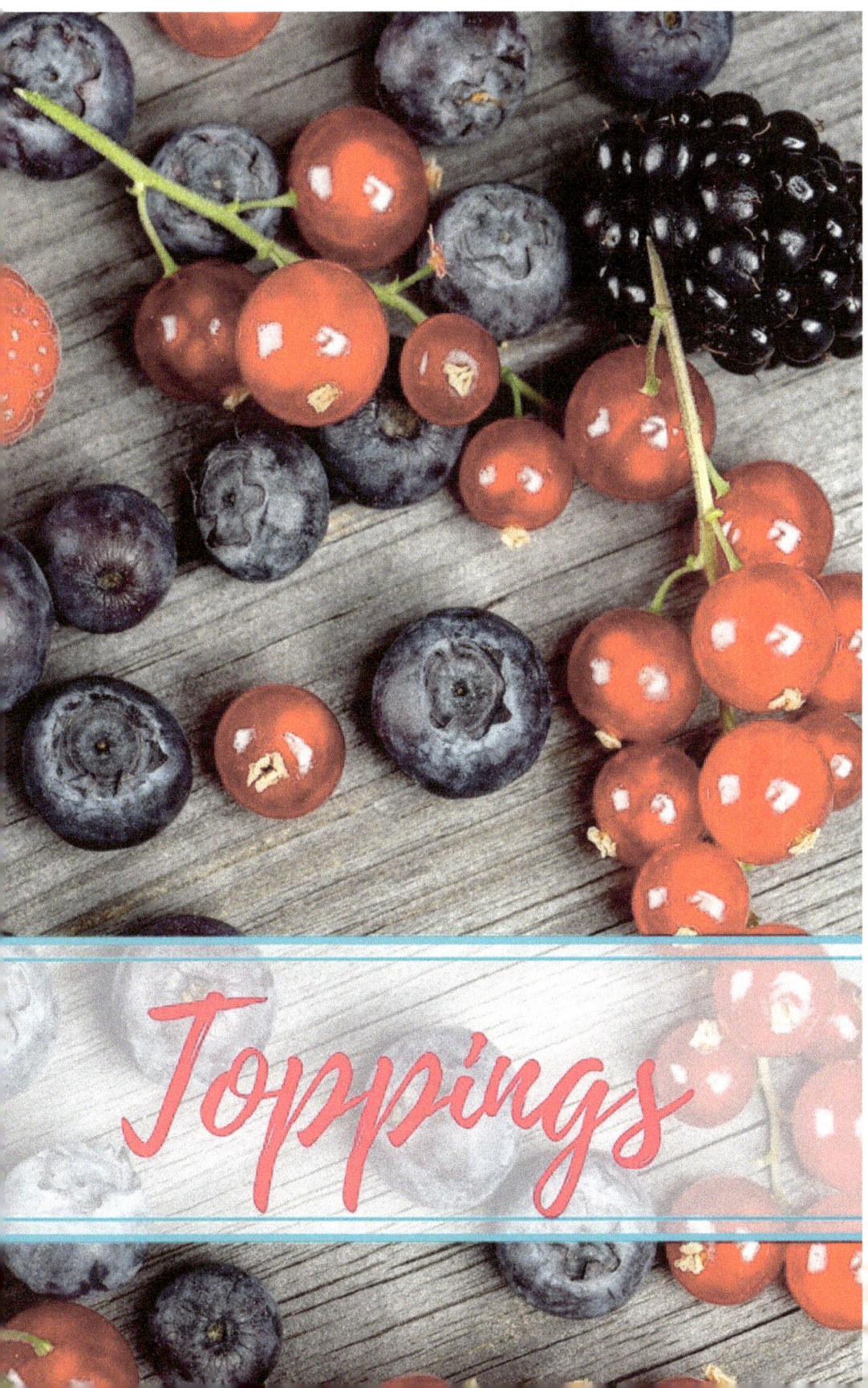

Berry Coulis

1/2 cup blueberries
1/2 cup raspberries
1/2 cup blackberries
1 tsp lemon juice

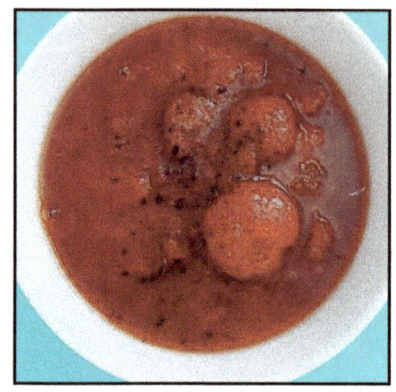

Procedure

1. Puree all ingredients in a Thermomix or high-speed blender until smooth.
2. Either cook in the Thermomix for 5 - 10 minutes until reduced and concentrated, or transfer to a small saucepan and complete this step.
3. Allow to cool slightly before adding to ice cream.
4. Unused portion can be stored in a sterilised glass jar in the refrigerator for up to one week.

Servings: 4

Preparation Time: 5 minutes

Cooking Time: 10 minutes

Total Time: 15 minutes

Nutrition Facts

Nutrition (per serving): 26 calories, <1g total fat, 0mg cholesterol, <1mg sodium, 67.6mg potassium, 6.3g carbohydrates, 2.4g fibre, 3.4g sugar, <1g protein.

Caramel Sauce

8 dates, pitted
1 cup boiling water
1 pinch salt

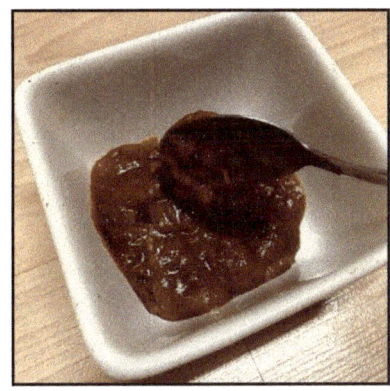

Procedure

1. Soak the dates boiling water for 5 - 10 minutes, then drain and remove skins.
2. Add dates and salt to a Thermomix or high-speed blender and blend for 2 - 4 minutes until smooth.
3. Allow to cool slightly before adding to ice cream.
4. Unused portion can be stored in a sterilised glass jar in the refrigerator for up to one week.

Servings: 4

Preparation Time: 10 minutes

Total Time: 10 minutes

Nutrition Facts

Nutrition (per serving): 133 calories, <1g total fat, 0mg cholesterol, 74.9mg sodium, 334.7mg potassium, 36g carbohydrates, 3.2g fibre, 31.9g sugar, <1g protein.

Caramel Sauce (Creamy)

300 mL coconut milk
1 tsp vanilla extract
1/2 tsp maple syrup
1 pinch salt

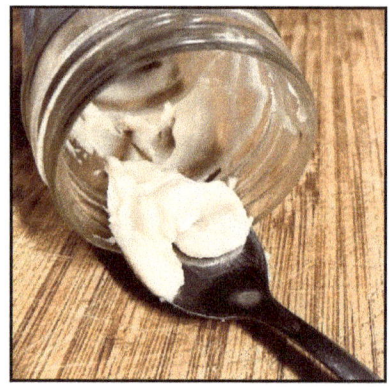

Procedure

1. Heat the coconut milk, salt and maple syrup in a saucepan, combine well.
2. Bring to the boil and boil for 3 - 4 minutes.
3. Reduce heat and simmer for a further 5 minutes, stirring occasionally.
4. Remove from heat and stir in vanilla, then allow to cool.
5. Unused portion can be stored in a sterilised glass jar in the refrigerator for up to one week.

Servings: 6

Preparation Time: 5 minutes

Cooking Time: 10 minutes

Total Time: 15 minutes

Nutrition Facts

Nutrition (per serving): 102 calories, 10.7g total fat, 0mg cholesterol, 55.1mg sodium, 112.2mg potassium, 1.9g carbohydrates, 0g fibre, <1g sugar, 1g protein.

Chocolate Sauce

1/2 cup coconut oil
1.5 tbsp cacao powder
1 tsp vanilla extract
1 tbsp maple syrup (optional)
1 pinch salt

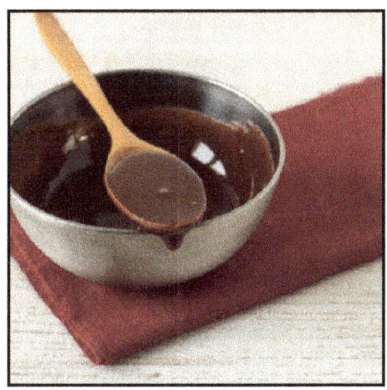

Procedure

1. Melt coconut oil in a saucepan over low heat.
2. Remove from heat and add salt and cacao, stirring constantly.
3. Add vanilla (and maple if using) and whisk with a fork or small whisk until smooth and glossy.
4. Allow to cool slightly before adding to ice cream.
5. Unused portion can be stored in a sterilised glass jar in the refrigerator for up to one week.

Servings: 6

Preparation Time: 10 minutes

Total Time: 10 minutes

Nutrition Facts

Nutrition (per serving): 170 calories, 18.3g total fat, 0mg cholesterol, 49.1mg sodium, 8.1mg potassium, 2.5g carbohydrates, <1g fibre, 2.4g sugar, <1g protein.

Recipe Tips

Change the flavour by adding food-grade essential oils such as orange, peppermint, grapefruit etc.
Add grated ginger, lemon rind or spices for a different flavour.

Peanut Butter Sauce

2 tbsp coconut oil

4 tbsp peanut butter (no added sugar)

1 tsp honey

1 tsp vanilla extract

1 pinch salt

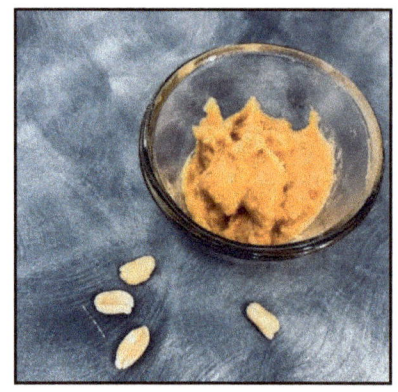

Procedure

1. Melt coconut oil in a saucepan over low heat.
2. Remove from heat and add peanut butter and salt, stirring constantly.
3. Allow to cool slightly before adding to ice cream.
4. Unused portion can be stored in a sterilised glass jar in the refrigerator for up to one week.

Servings: 6

Preparation Time: 10 minutes

Total Time: 10 minutes

Nutrition Facts

Nutrition (per serving): 104 calories, 9.9g total fat, 0mg cholesterol, 50.3mg sodium, 80.5mg potassium, 2.4g carbohydrates, <1g fibre, <1g sugar, 2.6g protein.

Recipe Tips

Change the flavour by adding food-grade essential oils such as orange, peppermint, grapefruit etc.
Add grated ginger, lemon rind or spices for a different flavour.

Strawberry Basil Sauce

1 punnet strawberries, washed and trimmed

1/2 tsp vanilla extract

1 sprig basil leaves, finely chopped

1 tsp lemon juice

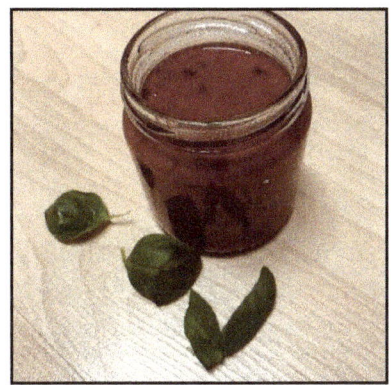

Procedure

1. Puree all ingredients in a Thermomix or high-speed blender until smooth.
2. Either cook in the Thermomix for 5 - 10 minutes until reduced and concentrated, or transfer to a small saucepan and complete this step.
3. Allow to cool slightly before adding to ice cream.
4. Unused portion can be stored in a sterilised glass jar in the refrigerator for up to one week.

Servings: 4

Preparation Time: 5 minutes

Cooking Time: 10 minutes

Total Time: 15 minutes

Nutrition Facts

Nutrition (per serving): 14 calories, <1g total fat, 0mg cholesterol, <1mg sodium, 64.1mg potassium, 3.1g carbohydrates, <1g fibre, 2g sugar, <1g protein.

Index

B

Banana 20
Berry Coulis 30
Berry Ice Cream 21

C

Caramel Sauce 31
Chai Cashew 7
Choc banana ice cream .. 22
Chocolate 11
Chocolate Coconut 23
Chocolate Sauce 33
Cinnamon Scroll 12
Coffee 13
Creamy Caramel Sauce . 32

G

Ginger and Cinnamon 14

L

Lemon 15

M

Mango 24
Matcha Green Tea 2
Mint Choc Chip 3

O

Orange 25

P

Peanut Butter Sauce 34
Peanut butter thunk 26
Pistachio 4

R

Rich Chocolate 5
Rum and Raisin Vanilla Bean 16

S

Salted Caramel 17
Strawberry Basil Ice cream 27
Strawberry Basil Sauce ... 35

T

Toasted Hazelnut and Coconut 8
Tropical Sorbet 28

V

Vanilla 9
Vanilla Bean 18

DM Plant Based Ice Cream

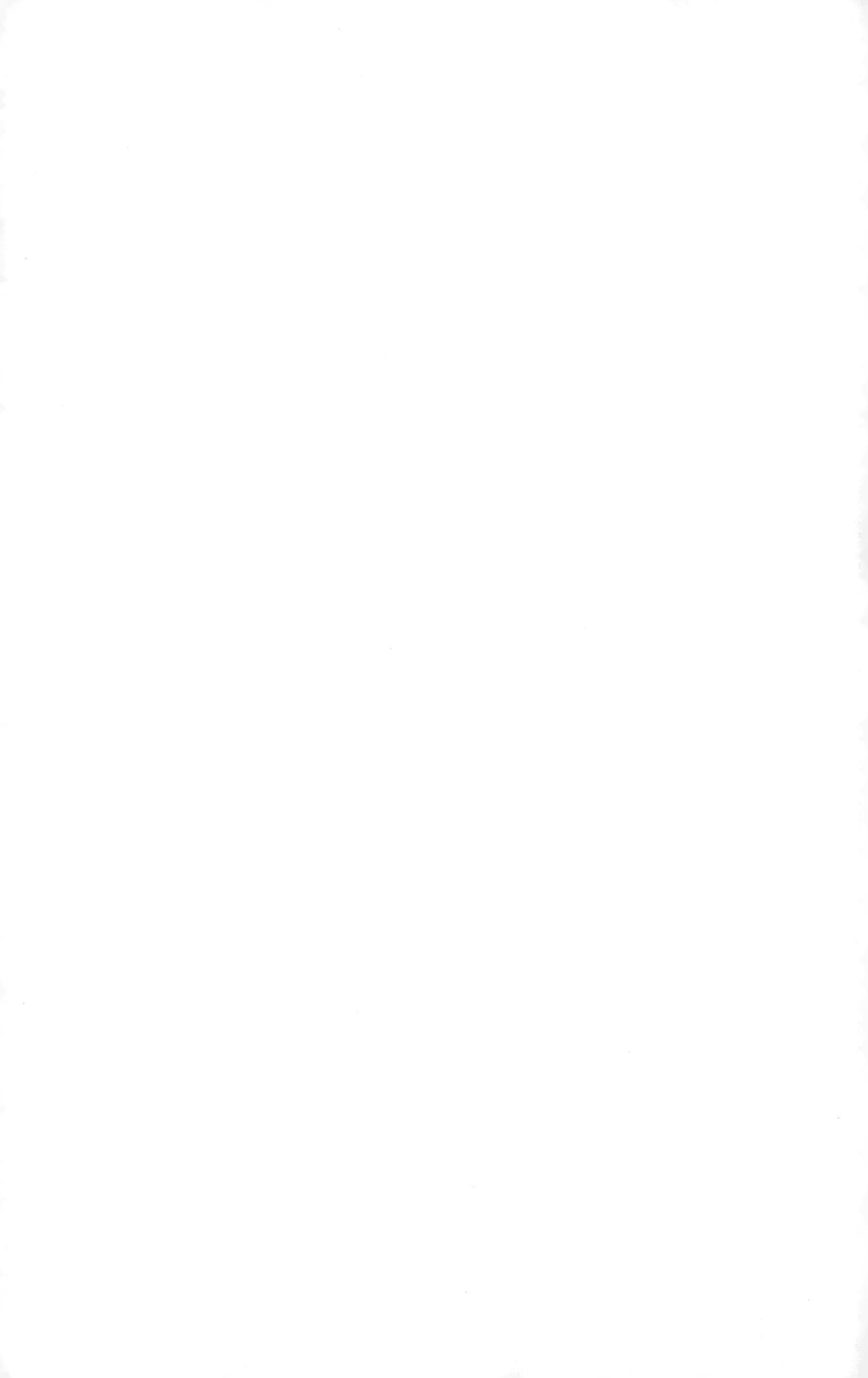

www.ingramcontent.com/pod-product-compliance
Lightning Source LLC
Chambersburg PA
CBHW062106290426
44110CB00022B/2731